How to Stop Sugar Cravings: The Ultimate guide Beat Sugar Addiction for Good

By Dr. Lucille Harris

Table of Content

Introduction

Sarah, trapped in the grip of sugar cravings, discovered a life-altering book on conquering addiction. Skeptical yet hopeful, she immersed herself in its pages. The book unveiled a wealth of knowledge, explaining the physiological and psychological aspects of cravings while offering practical strategies for control and healthier habits.

Embracing the book's wisdom, Sarah underwent a remarkable transformation. The once overpowering cravings lost their hold as she learned to satisfy her sweet tooth with wholesome, nutrient-rich foods. Her energy levels soared, and her mood stabilized.

The book's true power lay in empowering Sarah and others to reclaim their health and happiness. It became a beacon of hope, illuminating a path to freedom from sugar addiction. Ultimately, it not only curbed Sarah's cravings but also liberated her from the chains that held her back. It exemplified the transformative potential of knowledge and its profound impact on our lives.

Chapter One
Understanding Sugar addiction

Sugar addiction is a condition in which a person experiences a physical and psychological craving for sugar. This addiction is characterized by a need for frequent consumption of sugary foods and drinks, a lack of control over the amount of sugar intake, and continued use of sugar in spite of negative consequences.

Sugar addiction can be caused by a variety of factors, such as overeating, using sugar to cope with stress, and eating sugary foods as a reward. The symptoms of sugar addiction include cravings, irritability, headaches, fatigue, and difficulty concentrating.

Treatment options for sugar addiction can include diet and lifestyle modifications, counseling, and support groups. It is important to note that sugar addiction is not necessarily a sign of a deeper psychological issue; rather, it is a physical and psychological response to the consumption of sugar.

Reasons for Sugar Addiction

In the modern world, sugar has become an integral part of our daily lives. From sweet treats to processed foods, it seems nearly impossible to avoid its tempting allure. However, many individuals find themselves grappling with the powerful grip of sugar addiction, struggling to resist its cravings.

In this book, we aim to delve into the underlying reasons for sugar addiction, helping you understand the factors that contribute to these cravings and providing valuable insights to break free from their clutches.

1. Evolutionary Biology: Human beings have evolved to seek out and consume sweet-tasting foods. Our ancestors relied on high-calorie foods to survive periods of scarcity. As a result, the preference for sweetness became deeply ingrained in our biology. Unfortunately, in today's world of readily available sugary foods, this evolutionary adaptation can lead to addictive behaviors and unhealthy eating habits.

2. Brain Chemistry: Dopamine, a neurotransmitter linked to pleasure and reward, is released in the brain when sugar is consumed. The feeling of euphoria brought on by this release increases the desire to eat more sweets. As a result of the brain's gradual adaptation to these dopamine spikes, more sugar is needed to produce the same degree of satisfaction. This loop feeds the addiction and increases the need for sweet foods.

3. Emotional and Psychological Factors:
Sugar often becomes a source of comfort and emotional relief. Stress, anxiety, depression, and boredom can trigger a desire for sweet foods as a means of seeking temporary solace. Consuming sugar leads to a temporary mood elevation due to increased serotonin levels, giving individuals a momentary escape from negative emotions. However, this reliance on sugar as a coping mechanism can easily spiral into addiction.

4. Food Industry Marketing:
The food industry plays a significant role in promoting sugar addiction. Manufacturers intentionally create highly palatable products packed with sugar, salt, and unhealthy fats. Clever marketing techniques, vibrant packaging, and strategic product placement influence our buying decisions and perpetuate the desire for sugary foods. This constant exposure to enticing advertisements and easily accessible sugary snacks makes it challenging to resist cravings.

5. Habit Formation: Habits are powerful and can drive addictive behavior. When sugar is consumed regularly, the body becomes accustomed to its intake, leading to increased tolerance and dependency. Over time, the brain creates strong neural connections, associating specific situations, emotions, or environments with the consumption of sugar. Breaking these habits requires conscious effort and a willingness to adopt healthier alternatives.

6. Nutritional Deficiencies:
Deficiencies in essential nutrients like vitamins, minerals, and fiber can contribute to sugar cravings. Imbalances in blood sugar levels, caused by inadequate nutrition, can trigger intense urges for sugar. The body seeks quick energy sources, leading individuals to reach for sugary snacks as a rapid fix. Addressing these deficiencies through a balanced diet can help reduce cravings and support overall well-being.

Understanding the reasons behind sugar addiction is an essential step towards overcoming its grasp. By acknowledging the evolutionary, biological, emotional, psychological, and environmental factors that contribute to this addiction, individuals can take proactive measures to regain control over their health and well-being.

Benefits of Stopping Sugar Addiction

The pervasive presence of sugar in our modern diets has led to an alarming rise in sugar addiction. However, breaking free from this addiction can have transformative effects on both our physical and mental well-being. In this book, we explore the numerous benefits of stopping sugar addiction, providing you with the motivation and tools to embark on a healthier and more fulfilling lifestyle.

1. Increased Energy Levels: One of the immediate benefits of freeing yourself from sugar addiction is a significant boost in energy levels. Refined sugar causes blood sugar spikes followed by crashes, leaving you feeling tired and lethargic. By eliminating or reducing sugar intake, your energy levels stabilize, providing sustained vitality throughout the day. Say goodbye to those mid-afternoon slumps and embrace a renewed sense of vigor.

2. Weight Management and Improved Body Composition: Sugar-laden foods are often high in calories and lacking in nutritional value. By eliminating these empty calories, you can better manage your weight and improve your body composition.

Breaking free from sugar addiction allows you to focus on nutrient-dense foods, leading to healthier weight loss or maintenance. Shedding excess pounds not only enhances physical appearance but also reduces the risk of chronic diseases such as diabetes, heart disease, and certain types of cancer.

3. Enhanced Mental Clarity and Focus:

Excessive sugar consumption can negatively impact cognitive function, leading to brain fog and difficulty concentrating. By eliminating sugar, you can experience improved mental clarity and enhanced focus. Stable blood sugar levels support optimal brain function, allowing you to think more clearly, make better decisions, and perform tasks more efficiently. Say hello to improved productivity and a sharper mind.

4. Balanced Mood and Emotional Well-being:

Sugar addiction has a profound impact on mood and emotional stability. The rollercoaster effect of sugar on blood sugar levels can contribute to mood swings, irritability, and even symptoms of depression.

By breaking free from sugar addiction, you can achieve a more balanced mood and emotional well-being. Stable blood sugar levels promote the production of serotonin, the "feel-good" hormone, leading to a greater sense of happiness, contentment, and emotional resilience.

5. Improved Digestive Health: Excessive sugar consumption can wreak havoc on your digestive system. It feeds harmful gut bacteria, leading to imbalances and potential digestive issues such as bloating, gas, and constipation. Eliminating or reducing sugar allows the beneficial gut bacteria to thrive, promoting a healthier digestive system. You may experience improved bowel regularity, reduced inflammation, and a strengthened immune system.

6. Long-term Health Benefits: Stopping sugar addiction sets the stage for long-term health benefits. By reducing your intake of sugary foods, you lower your risk of developing chronic diseases such as type 2 diabetes, cardiovascular disease, obesity, and certain types of cancer. Taking control of your sugar consumption is a proactive step towards safeguarding your health and ensuring a higher quality of life as you age.

The benefits of breaking free from sugar addiction are far-reaching and encompass both physical and mental well-being. By reclaiming control over your diet and reducing sugar consumption, you can experience increased energy, improved weight management, enhanced mental clarity, balanced mood, better digestive health, and long-term protection against chronic diseases.

Chapter Two
Understanding the Problem

Sugar addiction has become a pervasive problem in today's society, affecting individuals of all ages and backgrounds. To effectively address this issue and embark on the path to recovery, it is crucial to gain a comprehensive understanding of the complexities surrounding sugar addiction. In this book, we delve deep into the roots of the problem, unraveling the various factors that contribute to sugar addiction and equipping you with the knowledge necessary to overcome its challenges.

1. The Addictive Nature of Sugar: Sugar addiction is more than just a lack of self-control or willpower. The effect sugar has on the brain is what makes it so addicting. Dopamine, a neurotransmitter linked to pleasure and reward, is released after consuming sugar. The exhilaration brought on by this release increases the craving for sugar. The dopamine response in the brain gradually gets desensitized, which increases the desire for more sugar to satiate the same level of satisfaction. It is easier to comprehend the strong effects that sugar may have on our bodies and thoughts when we are aware of the neurochemical processes at work.

2. Hidden and Pervasive Nature of Sugar: Sugar is not only present in obvious sources such as sweets and sugary beverages but also hides in numerous processed foods and condiments. Manufacturers often add sugar to enhance flavor and extend shelf life. This pervasive presence makes it challenging to avoid sugar completely, as it lurks in unexpected places like sauces, salad dressings, and even seemingly healthy foods like yogurt or granola bars. Recognizing the hidden sources of sugar empowers us to make informed choices and navigate the food landscape more effectively.

3. Emotional and Psychological Triggers: Sugar addiction often intertwines with emotional and psychological triggers. Many individuals turn to sugary foods as a form of comfort or stress relief, using them as a coping mechanism to deal with negative emotions or situations. Sugar temporarily boosts serotonin levels, offering a momentary escape from stress, anxiety, or sadness. Identifying the emotional and psychological factors that drive sugar cravings is crucial in developing healthier coping mechanisms and breaking the cycle of addiction.

4. Societal and Cultural Factors: Societal and cultural factors play a significant role in shaping our relationship with sugar. Advertisements, food marketing, and social norms influence our choices and attitudes towards sugary foods. The prevalence of convenience foods, fast food chains, and the abundance of sugary snacks contribute to the normalization of excessive sugar consumption. Recognizing the impact of societal and cultural influences allows us to challenge and reshape our perceptions and behaviors surrounding sugar.

5. Habit Formation and Environmental Triggers: Habits play a substantial role in perpetuating sugar addiction. The repeated consumption of sugar establishes strong neural connections in the brain, associating certain situations, environments, or emotions with the desire for sugary foods. Additionally, environmental triggers such as the sight or smell of sugary treats can intensify cravings. Understanding the power of habit formation and environmental triggers equips us with strategies to break free from the cycle of addiction.

Gaining a deep understanding of the complexities surrounding sugar addiction is a vital step towards recovery and long-term success. By recognizing the addictive nature of sugar, identifying hidden sources, acknowledging emotional and psychological triggers, understanding societal influences, and addressing habit formation, we can develop effective strategies to overcome sugar addiction.

The Brain and Sugar Addiction

Sugar addiction is not simply a matter of willpower or self-control. It is deeply rooted in the intricate workings of the brain. Understanding the neurological mechanisms behind sugar addiction is key to breaking free from its grip. In this book, we delve into the fascinating world of the brain and its relationship with sugar, unraveling the intricate processes that contribute to addiction and offering insights to reclaim control over your cravings.

1. The Reward System: Dopamine and Pleasure At the heart of sugar addiction lies the brain's reward system. When we consume sugar, it stimulates the release of dopamine, a neurotransmitter associated with pleasure and reward. Dopamine creates a sense of euphoria, reinforcing the desire to seek out more sugar. Over time, the brain adapts to the constant dopamine spikes, leading to tolerance and cravings for higher sugar doses. Understanding this reward system helps us comprehend why sugar can have such a powerful hold on our behavior.

2. Sugar and the Brain's Craving Pathways: Sugar addiction affects the brain's craving pathways, which are responsible for generating intense desires for certain substances or experiences. Consuming sugar activates these pathways, creating a cycle of craving and reward. The more sugar we consume, the stronger the cravings become. These pathways, involving regions such as the prefrontal cortex, amygdala, and striatum, establish neural connections that contribute to the persistence of sugar addiction.

3, Hijacked Brain: Similarities with Drug Addiction
Research suggests that sugar addiction shares similarities with substance abuse disorders, such as drug addiction. Studies using brain imaging techniques have shown overlapping neurological responses between sugar and drugs like cocaine or opioids. The repeated consumption of sugar can lead to neuroadaptations, altering brain circuits and reinforcing addictive behaviors. Recognizing these parallels helps us comprehend the seriousness of sugar addiction and the importance of addressing it as a significant health concern.

4. Cravings and Withdrawal Symptoms: Sugar addiction can induce powerful cravings and withdrawal symptoms when consumption is reduced or eliminated. The brain becomes accustomed to the constant presence of sugar and adjusts its functioning accordingly. When sugar intake is reduced, the brain reacts by signaling cravings and triggering uncomfortable symptoms such as irritability, mood swings, headaches, and fatigue. Understanding these withdrawal symptoms as part of the addiction process empowers individuals to persevere through the initial challenges and reach a healthier state.

5. Neuroplasticity and Breaking the Cycle: The brain's remarkable ability to change and adapt, known as neuroplasticity, offers hope for overcoming sugar addiction. By intentionally rewiring neural connections and creating new habits, we can break free from the addictive cycle. Engaging in healthier behaviors, adopting mindful eating practices, and retraining the brain's response to sugar can help weaken the cravings and reestablish control. Understanding the brain's capacity for change provides optimism and motivation on the path to recovery.

The brain's intricate workings play a fundamental role in sugar addiction. From the reward system and craving pathways to the similarities with drug addiction and the potential for neuroplasticity, understanding the brain's involvement empowers individuals to regain control over their cravings.

By comprehending the neurological processes at play, we can develop strategies and interventions to break free from sugar addiction, leading to improved overall health and well-being.

The Effects of Sugar Addiction

Sugar addiction goes beyond momentary pleasure; its detrimental effects can impact both our physical and mental well-being. Understanding these effects is crucial in recognizing the urgency of breaking free from sugar addiction. In this book, we explore the profound impact of sugar addiction on various aspects of our health, shedding light on the consequences it has on our mind, body, and overall quality of life.

1. Weight Gain and Obesity: Excessive sugar consumption is a leading contributor to weight gain and obesity. Sugary foods are often calorie-dense and lack nutritional value. Regularly consuming these empty calories leads to an imbalance between energy intake and expenditure, resulting in weight gain. Furthermore, the high-fructose corn syrup found in many sugary products can disrupt hunger-regulating hormones, leading to increased appetite and overeating.

2. Increased Risk of Chronic Diseases: Sugar addiction has been linked to a higher risk of developing chronic diseases. Excessive sugar intake can lead to insulin resistance, a precursor to type 2 diabetes. It also contributes to inflammation, which is implicated in the development of various diseases, including heart disease, stroke, and certain types of cancer. By breaking free from sugar addiction, individuals can mitigate these risks and improve their long-term health outcomes.

3. Dental Health Problems: Sugar is a major contributor to tooth decay and dental health issues. Bacteria in the mouth feed on sugar, producing acids that erode tooth enamel and lead to cavities. Frequent sugar consumption increases the likelihood of dental caries and gum disease, compromising oral health. By reducing sugar intake, individuals can protect their teeth and gums, promoting better dental hygiene.

4. Energy Fluctuations and Fatigue: While sugar provides a quick burst of energy, it often leads to subsequent crashes and fatigue. Refined sugar causes rapid spikes in blood sugar levels, followed by sharp drops. These fluctuations can result in feelings of tiredness, lethargy, and difficulty concentrating. Breaking free from sugar addiction allows for more stable energy levels throughout the day, promoting sustained vitality and improved cognitive function.

5. Mood Swings and Mental Health Issues: Sugar addiction can have a significant impact on mental health and emotional well-being. The rollercoaster effect of sugar on blood sugar levels can contribute to mood swings, irritability, and increased anxiety. Moreover, excessive sugar consumption has been associated with an increased risk of depression and a higher likelihood of developing mental health disorders. By reducing sugar intake, individuals may experience improved mood stability and enhanced mental resilience.

6. Skin Problems and Aging: Sugar can have adverse effects on skin health and contribute to premature aging. High sugar consumption can lead to glycation, a process where sugar molecules attach to proteins, causing the formation of harmful compounds that damage collagen and elastin fibers.

This process accelerates skin aging, leading to wrinkles, sagging, and a dull complexion. By curbing sugar addiction, individuals can support healthier, more youthful-looking skin.

The effects of sugar addiction extend far beyond momentary indulgence. They encompass weight gain, increased risk of chronic diseases, dental health problems, energy fluctuations, mood swings, mental health issues, and skin problems. Recognizing the toll sugar addiction takes on our mind and body is a crucial step towards reclaiming our health and well-being.

Physical and Mental Health Concerns

Sugar addiction can have far-reaching consequences, not only on our physical well-being but also on our mental health. Understanding the physical and mental health concerns associated with sugar addiction is essential for taking proactive steps towards breaking free from its grip. In this book, we delve into the intricate relationship between sugar addiction and its impact on our physical and mental well-being, empowering individuals to make informed choices for a healthier and more balanced life.

Physical Health Concerns:

a) Weight Gain and Obesity: Excessive sugar consumption contributes to weight gain and obesity. Sugary foods are often high in calories and provide little nutritional value. Over time, the accumulation of excess body fat can lead to various health issues such as cardiovascular disease, diabetes, and joint problems.

b) Type 2 Diabetes: Sugar addiction increases the risk of developing type 2 diabetes. Consistently high sugar intake can lead to insulin resistance, impairing the body's ability to regulate blood sugar levels effectively. Over time, this can progress to diabetes, a chronic condition associated with numerous complications.

c) Cardiovascular Health: Sugar addiction can negatively impact cardiovascular health. High sugar intake has been linked to an increased risk of heart disease, high blood pressure, and abnormal lipid profiles. It contributes to inflammation and oxidative stress, damaging blood vessels and promoting the development of atherosclerosis.

d) Dental Issues: Excessive sugar consumption contributes to tooth decay and dental cavities. Sugar feeds harmful bacteria in the mouth, leading to acid production and enamel erosion. This can result in tooth decay, gum disease, and oral health problems.

Mental Health Concerns

a) **Mood Disorders:** Sugar addiction can influence mood and exacerbate mood disorders such as anxiety and depression. The rapid spikes and crashes in blood sugar levels can lead to mood swings, irritability, and fatigue. Long-term sugar addiction may disrupt the balance of neurotransmitters in the brain, contributing to emotional instability.

b) **Cognitive Function:** High sugar consumption has been associated with impaired cognitive function and an increased risk of cognitive decline. Studies have shown that sugar addiction may negatively affect memory, learning, and attention span. The inflammatory effects of excessive sugar intake can also impact brain health and increase the risk of neurodegenerative disorders.

c) Addiction and Reward Pathways: Sugar addiction shares commonalities with substance addiction in terms of the brain's reward pathways. Over time, the brain becomes desensitized to the effects of sugar, leading to cravings and a desire for higher doses to achieve the same level of satisfaction. This can contribute to addictive behaviors and a cycle of dependency.

d) Mental Well-being: Sugar addiction can affect overall mental well-being and self-esteem. The negative consequences of sugar consumption, such as weight gain and poor physical health, can lead to feelings of guilt, shame, and lowered self-confidence. Breaking free from sugar addiction can improve self-image and promote a more positive mental outlook.

The physical and mental health concerns associated with sugar addiction are significant and wide-ranging.

From weight gain and obesity to diabetes, cardiovascular issues, dental problems, mood disorders, cognitive impairment, and addiction-like behaviors, sugar addiction takes a toll on both our bodies and minds. Recognizing these concerns is the first step towards breaking free from sugar addiction and adopting a healthier lifestyle.

Chapter Three
Strategies for Overcoming Sugar Addiction

Overcoming sugar addiction can be a challenging journey, but with the right strategies and tools, it is entirely possible to break free from its grip. In this book, we provide you with a comprehensive guide to help you navigate the path to recovery and empower you to take charge of your health. By implementing effective strategies, you can overcome cravings, develop healthier habits, and achieve a life free from the clutches of sugar addiction.

1. Understand and Educate Yourself: Knowledge is power when it comes to overcoming sugar addiction. Educate yourself about the detrimental effects of excessive sugar consumption on your physical and mental well-being. Learn about the hidden sources of sugar in foods and the impact it has on your body. Understanding the reasons behind your addiction will help you build motivation and reinforce your commitment to change.

2. Set Clear and Realistic Goals: Establish clear and achievable goals to guide your journey towards overcoming sugar addiction. Define specific targets such as reducing daily sugar intake, eliminating sugary beverages, or avoiding processed foods high in added sugars. Ensure your goals are realistic and sustainable, allowing for gradual progress rather than drastic changes that may lead to feelings of deprivation or failure.

3. Identify and Replace Triggers: Recognize the triggers that lead to your sugar cravings. These triggers can be emotional, environmental, or habitual. Keep a journal to track your cravings and identify patterns. Once you have identified your triggers, develop alternative strategies to cope with them. For example, engage in stress-relieving activities like exercise or mindfulness meditation, remove sugary foods from your environment, or replace sugary snacks with healthier options like fruits or nuts.

4. Practice Mindful Eating: Adopt mindful eating practices to enhance your awareness of your food choices and eating habits. Pay attention to hunger and fullness cues, and savor each bite of your meals. Slow down the eating process, focusing on the flavors, textures, and nourishment that food provides. This helps you develop a more conscious relationship with food and reduces the likelihood of mindless sugar consumption.

5. Plan and Make Nutritious Meals: Take charge of your diet by organizing and making healthy meals ahead of time. Make a meal plan that places a focus on nutrient-dense, whole foods. Your meals should contain a variety of fruits, vegetables, lean proteins, complete grains, and healthy fats. You can lessen the temptation to go for sugary snacks or convenience foods by having healthy options close at hand.

6. Find Healthy Substitutes: Discover and experiment with healthy substitutes for sugary foods and beverages. Satisfy your sweet tooth with naturally sweet alternatives like fresh fruits, dates, or stevia. Opt for unsweetened beverages such as herbal teas, infused water, or sparkling water. Gradually train your taste buds to appreciate the natural sweetness of foods without relying on added sugars.

7. Seek Support and Accountability: Enlist the support of friends, family, or a support group who understand your journey and share similar goals. Share your struggles, successes, and progress with them, and lean on their encouragement and guidance. Having a support system provides accountability, motivation, and a safe space to share your experiences and challenges.

8. Celebrate Non-Food Rewards: Reframe your mindset around rewards and find non-food ways to treat yourself. Instead of using sugary treats as a reward, indulge in activities you enjoy, such as a spa day, a movie night, a new book, or spending quality time with loved ones. Celebrate your achievements in ways that nourish your soul and promote self-care.

Overcoming sugar addiction requires determination, commitment, and the implementation of effective strategies. By understanding the underlying causes of your addiction, setting realistic goals, identifying triggers, practicing mindful eating, planning and preparing healthy meals, finding healthy substitutes, seeking support and accountability, and celebrating non-food rewards, you can break free from the grip of sugar addiction and reclaim control over your health and well-being.

Remember that the journey to overcoming sugar addiction is a process that may have ups and downs.On your journey, practice patience and self-kindness. Celebrate every small victory and learn from any setbacks. With perseverance and a willingness to embrace healthier habits, you can transform your relationship with sugar and enjoy a life filled with vitality, balance, and overall well-being.

By implementing these strategies and making a conscious effort to change your habits, you can overcome sugar addiction and embark on a journey towards a healthier and happier life. Take the first step today and embrace the possibilities that lie ahead. You have the power to break free from sugar's hold and create a future filled with vitality and optimal health.

Establishing a Routine

Establishing a routine is a powerful tool in overcoming sugar addiction. By creating structure and consistency in your daily life, you can build healthy habits, reinforce positive behaviors, and minimize the temptation to indulge in sugary foods. In this book, we explore the importance of establishing a routine and provide practical guidance on how to implement and maintain a routine that supports your journey towards overcoming sugar addiction.

1. Set Clear Goals and Priorities: Set priorities and goals for your sugar addiction journey right now. Describe your goals and why they are important to you. You can use these objectives as a compass to direct your routine and maintain your motivation. Put your health and wellbeing first, and let that direct your choices and deeds.

2. Design Your Ideal Routine: Consider your lifestyle, responsibilities, and personal preferences to design a routine that works for you. Identify the times of day when you are most likely to experience cravings or vulnerability to sugar, and plan activities that can help distract or redirect your focus during those times. Include time for meal planning, physical activity, self-care, and engaging in activities that bring you joy and fulfillment.

3. Establish Consistent Meal Times: Regular and consistent meal times can help stabilize your blood sugar levels and reduce cravings. Plan and prepare balanced meals that include a variety of whole foods to provide sustained energy and nutrition throughout the day. Avoid skipping meals, as it can lead to blood sugar fluctuations and increase the likelihood of reaching for sugary snacks.

4. Create a Balanced Plate: Consider producing a balanced plate with a range of nutrients when planning your meals. Include a lot of fruits and vegetables, complex carbohydrates, lean proteins, healthy fats, and complex carbohydrates. You'll feel nourished and satiated thanks to this balance, which will lessen your craving for sweets.

5. Incorporate Physical Activity: Regular physical activity is an essential component of overcoming sugar addiction. Include exercise or movement in your routine to support your overall well-being. Find activities that you enjoy, such as walking, dancing, yoga, or strength training. Engaging in physical activity not only helps distract from cravings but also releases endorphins, improves mood, and boosts energy levels.

6. Schedule Time for Self-Care: Self-care is essential for stress management and preserving a positive outlook. Make self-care activities that allow you to unwind and refresh a priority. This could involve engaging in activities that make you happy, such as reading, listening to music, taking relaxing baths, practicing mindfulness or meditation. By taking care of your emotional needs, you lessen the possibility of using sugar as a comfort or stress reliever.

7. Plan for Healthy Snacks: Prepare and keep healthy snacks readily available to combat cravings and prevent impulsive choices. Stock your pantry and fridge with nutritious options such as cut-up fruits, vegetables with hummus, unsalted nuts, Greek yogurt, or homemade energy bars. When hunger strikes between meals, reach for these healthier alternatives instead of reaching for sugary snacks.

8. Get Sufficient Sleep: Adequate sleep is crucial for overall health and helps regulate hormones that impact appetite and cravings. Establish a consistent sleep schedule that allows for 7-9 hours of quality sleep each night. Create a bedtime routine that promotes relaxation and signals to your body that it's time to rest.

9. Stay Hydrated: Sometimes hunger or urges are misinterpreted for dehydration. Aim to consume enough water each day by keeping a water bottle on you at all times. Drinking plenty of water helps improve digestion, boost overall health, and lessen cravings for sweet drinks.

10. Evaluate and Adjust: Examine your routine frequently to determine what is working well and what might need to be adjusted. Be adaptable and prepared to alter as necessary. Pay attention to how your routine is impacting your cravings, mood, and overall well-being. If certain activities or habits are triggering cravings or not aligning with your goals, modify them accordingly. Remember that creating a routine is an ongoing process of self-discovery and adaptation.

11. Stay Accountable: Establishing a routine requires accountability. Find a system of support that can act as a check on you and a source of inspiration. This could be a buddy, relative, or a group of supporters. Tell them about your objectives and developments, and enlist their help in staying on course.

12. Practice Patience and Persistence: Establishing a routine takes time and effort. It's important to practice patience and persistence as you navigate the journey of overcoming sugar addiction. Recognize that there may be setbacks or challenges along the way, but don't let them discourage you. Hold fast to your objectives and have faith in the process. Your habit will become more ingrained each day, making it simpler to withstand sugar cravings and make better decisions.

Establishing a routine is a valuable strategy in overcoming sugar addiction. By setting clear goals, designing a routine that supports your well-being, and incorporating healthy habits such as consistent meal times, balanced nutrition, physical activity, self-care, and proper sleep, you can create a structure that promotes long-term success.

Regular evaluation, adjustment, and accountability will ensure that your routine remains effective and aligned with your goals. Embrace the power of routine on your journey to breaking free from sugar addiction and embracing a healthier, more fulfilling life.

Reducing Exposure to Triggers

Reducing exposure to triggers is a crucial step in overcoming sugar addiction. Triggers are environmental, emotional, or situational cues that stimulate cravings and temptations for sugary foods. By identifying and minimizing exposure to these triggers, individuals can effectively manage their cravings, make healthier choices, and successfully navigate the path to breaking free from sugar addiction. In this book, we explore practical strategies for reducing exposure to triggers and regaining control over your relationship with sugar.

1. Identify Personal Triggers: Determine your unique sugar hunger triggers first. Think about the circumstances, feelings, or environments that influence your propensity to eat sugary foods. Stress, boredom, social gatherings, particular locations or activities, and particular times of the day are a few examples of common triggers. Understanding your triggers will help you take proactive steps to lessen their impact on your decisions.

2. Modify Your Environment: Create an environment that supports your goals of reducing sugar consumption. Clear your pantry and refrigerator of sugary snacks and beverages, replacing them with healthier alternatives. Keep your home stocked with fresh fruits, vegetables, nuts, and other nutritious options. By removing tempting sugary foods from your immediate surroundings, you reduce the likelihood of indulging in them.

3. Plan Ahead: Before attending social events or outings, plan ahead to minimize exposure to triggers. If you anticipate that sugary treats will be present, eat a balanced meal beforehand to reduce hunger and temptation. Bring your own healthy snacks or contribute a sugar-free dish to share. By being prepared, you can navigate social situations with confidence and resist the urge to consume sugary foods.

4. Practice Mindful Eating: Engage in mindful eating to reduce exposure to triggers and develop a healthier relationship with food. Slow down and savor each bite, paying attention to flavors, textures, and sensations. By being fully present during meals, you can better recognize feelings of satisfaction and prevent overeating or seeking sugary foods for emotional comfort.

5. Manage Stress: Sugar cravings are frequently triggered by stress. Create efficient stress management strategies to lessen the influence of stress on your decisions. Practice relaxing and stress-relieving activities, such as yoga, deep breathing exercises, meditation, or relaxing pastimes. Finding good coping mechanisms for stress will lessen the propensity to reach for sugary foods as a quick fix.

6. Seek Support: Enlist the support of family, friends, or a support group who understand your journey and share similar goals. Communicate your commitment to reducing sugar consumption and ask for their support in minimizing triggers. Having a support system can provide encouragement, accountability, and alternative strategies to navigate challenging situations.

7. Practice Emotional Awareness: Cravings for sugar are frequently influenced by emotional stimuli. Accurately recognize your emotions and control them. Create healthy coping strategies like writing, talking to a therapist or trusted friend, or doing things that make you feel better. You can lessen your dependency on sugary foods as a source of emotional comfort by addressing underlying feelings.

8. Create New Habits: Replace old habits that involve sugary foods with healthier alternatives. For example, if you typically reach for a sugary snack when feeling bored, find a new activity to engage in, such as going for a walk, practicing a hobby, or reading a book. By consciously creating new habits, you redirect your focus away from sugar and towards activities that promote your well-being.

9. Practice Self-Care: Engage in regular self-care activities to nourish your mind and body. Self-care reduces stress levels and promotes overall well-being, reducing the likelihood of turning to sugar for emotional comfort.

Engage in activities such as taking baths, practicing mindfulness or meditation, getting enough sleep, spending time in nature, and engaging in hobbies or activities that bring you joy. Prioritize self-care in your daily routine, and make time for activities that replenish your energy and help you relax.

10. Practice Assertiveness: Learn to assertively communicate your boundaries and preferences when it comes to food choices. If you're in a social setting where sugary foods are being offered, politely decline or opt for healthier options. Remember that it's okay to prioritize your health and well-being, even if it means deviating from social norms or expectations.

11. Keep a Trigger Journal: Maintain a trigger journal to track your cravings and identify patterns. Whenever you experience a sugar craving, write down the date, time, location, emotions, and any specific triggers that may have contributed to the craving. Over time, you'll start to notice trends and gain insight into the specific triggers that are most influential for you. This awareness will empower you to develop targeted strategies for managing those triggers effectively.

12. Celebrate Progress: Acknowledge and celebrate your progress along the way. Breaking free from sugar addiction is a journey, and every small step forward is worth celebrating. Reward yourself with non-food treats for reaching milestones or achieving personal goals. By acknowledging your achievements, you reinforce positive behaviors and build confidence in your ability to overcome sugar addiction.

Reducing exposure to triggers is an essential step in overcoming sugar addiction. By identifying personal triggers, modifying your environment, planning ahead, practicing mindful eating, managing stress, seeking support, practicing emotional awareness, creating new habits, prioritizing self-care, practicing assertiveness, keeping a trigger journal, and celebrating progress, you can effectively reduce the influence of triggers and regain control over your food choices.

Remember, breaking free from sugar addiction is a process that requires patience, self-compassion, and persistence. By implementing these strategies, you are taking an important step towards a healthier, happier, and more balanced life.

Eating Healthier Alternatives

When overcoming sugar addiction, finding healthier alternatives to satisfy your cravings is essential. By incorporating nutrient-dense and wholesome foods into your diet, you can nourish your body, support your overall health, and reduce your dependence on sugary treats. In this book, we explore a variety of delicious and nutritious alternatives that can help you break free from the grip of sugar addiction and create a healthier relationship with food.

1. Embrace Whole Foods: Place a priority on including complete, unadulterated foods in your diet. Fruits, vegetables, whole grains, lean meats, and healthy fats are a few of these. Essential nutrients, fiber, and antioxidants are found in whole foods, which can help control blood sugar levels, boost fullness, and lessen cravings.

2. Enjoy Fresh Fruits: Satisfy your sweet tooth with the natural sweetness of fresh fruits. Fruits contain natural sugars along with vitamins, minerals, and dietary fiber. Opt for a variety of colorful fruits such as berries, apples, oranges, and melons. They can be enjoyed on their own, added to smoothies, or used as toppings for yogurt or oatmeal.

3. Incorporate Healthy Fats: To improve flavor and encourage satiety, incorporate healthy fats into your diet. Olive oil, almonds, seeds, and avocados are great sources of good fats. Essential fatty acids are provided by these meals, which can also aid to normalize blood sugar levels and lessen cravings for sweets.

4. Choose Whole Grains: Replace refined grains with whole grains to provide sustained energy and improve nutritional value. Whole grains, such as quinoa, brown rice, whole wheat bread, and oats, are rich in fiber, vitamins, and minerals. They digest more slowly, preventing blood sugar spikes and maintaining a feeling of fullness.

5. Experiment with Natural Sweeteners: Instead of refined sugars, experiment with natural sweeteners that offer flavor without the negative effects of sugar. Stevia, monk fruit, and erythritol are low-calorie sweeteners that can be used in moderation. Additionally, spices like cinnamon, nutmeg, and vanilla extract can add natural sweetness to foods without adding sugar.

6. Discover Sugar-Free Snacks: Explore the wide range of sugar-free snacks available in the market. Look for snacks made with natural ingredients and sweetened with alternatives like stevia or monk fruit. Examples include sugar-free granola bars, dark chocolate with high cocoa content, and sugar-free nut butter spreads.

7. Indulge in Dark Chocolate: If you're craving chocolate, reach for dark chocolate with a high percentage of cocoa (70% or higher). Dark chocolate is lower in sugar and rich in antioxidants. It can satisfy your sweet tooth while providing potential health benefits.

8. Whip Up Healthy Treats: Get creative in the kitchen and experiment with homemade, healthier versions of your favorite treats. Look for recipes that use natural sweeteners, whole grain flours, and healthier fats. There are countless recipes available for sugar-free desserts, energy balls, and baked goods that can be enjoyed guilt-free.

9. Stay Hydrated: Often, we mistake thirst for hunger or sugar cravings. Stay hydrated throughout the day by drinking water, herbal teas, or infused water with fruits and herbs. Proper hydration can help reduce cravings and support overall well-being.

10. Practice Portion Control: While switching to healthier options can be advantageous, it's crucial to use portion control. Even more nutritious foods still have calories, and eating too much can lead to weight gain and other health problems. Pay attention to portion sizes and your body's signals of hunger and fullness.

Eating healthier alternatives is a key aspect of overcoming sugar addiction. By embracing whole foods, enjoying fresh fruits, incorporating healthy fats, choosing whole grains, experimenting with natural sweeteners, discovering sugar-free snacks, indulging in dark chocolate, whipping up healthy treats, staying hydrated, and practicing portion control, you can nourish your body without relying on sugar-laden foods.

These alternatives provide essential nutrients, satisfy your cravings, and support your overall health and well-being. Remember, breaking free from sugar addiction is a journey, and it requires patience, persistence, and a commitment to making positive changes in your diet.

By incorporating these healthier alternatives into your lifestyle, you can create a sustainable and enjoyable approach to eating that promotes long-term success and a balanced relationship with food. Say goodbye to sugar addiction and hello to a healthier, more vibrant you.

Boosting Self-Control

Self-control plays a vital role in overcoming sugar addiction. It enables you to resist temptations, make healthier choices, and maintain long-term success in your journey towards breaking free from the grip of sugar. In this book, we explore effective strategies and techniques to boost your self-control and empower you to regain control over your relationship with sugar.

1. Set Clear and Realistic Goals: Establish clear and realistic goals for reducing your sugar intake. Having a specific target in mind provides you with a sense of direction and purpose. Make your goals measurable and time-bound, which allows you to track your progress and celebrate milestones along the way.

2. Develop Awareness and Mindfulness: Cultivate awareness and mindfulness around your eating habits. Pay attention to your thoughts, emotions, and physical sensations when faced with sugary temptations. By being aware of the triggers and patterns that lead to cravings, you can respond in a more conscious and intentional manner.

3. Practice Delayed Gratification: Train yourself to delay gratification when it comes to sugar. Instead of giving in to immediate cravings, practice waiting and gradually reducing your intake over time. This strengthens your self-control muscle and helps break the cycle of instant gratification associated with sugar addiction.

4. Build a Supportive Environment: Surround yourself with a supportive environment that promotes your goals. Inform your friends and family about your journey to overcome sugar addiction, and ask for their support. Create an environment at home and work that is free from sugary temptations and filled with healthier alternatives.

5. Utilize Cognitive Restructuring: Challenge and reframe your thoughts and beliefs about sugar. Recognize the negative impact it has on your health and well-being. Replace thoughts like "I need sugar" with empowering affirmations such as "I choose nourishing foods that support my health and energy levels."

6. Implement Stress Management Techniques: Stress can undermine self-control and increase the likelihood of succumbing to sugar cravings. Explore stress management techniques such as deep breathing exercises, meditation, journaling, or engaging in physical activity. Find what works best for you to reduce stress levels and enhance your self-control.

7. Develop Healthy Coping Mechanisms: Find alternative, healthy ways to cope with emotions and stress rather than turning to sugar for comfort. Engage in activities that bring you joy, such as hobbies, spending time in nature, listening to music, or practicing self-care. Develop a toolbox of strategies that support your emotional well-being without relying on sugary foods.

8. Practice Self-Reflection: Regularly reflect on your progress and challenges along your journey to overcoming sugar addiction. Determine which tactics are effective and what needs to be improved. Celebrate your victories, take lessons from your failures, and modify your strategy as necessary. Self-reflection improves self-awareness and aids in future decision-making.

9. Boost Willpower with Proper Sleep: Adequate sleep is essential for maintaining willpower and self-control. Each night, try to get seven to eight hours of good sleep. Lack of sleep can affect how your hormones are regulated, lead to more cravings, and make it harder to resist temptation. Put sleep first as part of your overall plan for improving self-control.

Practice Self-Care and Stress Reduction: Engage in regular self-care activities to nurture your physical and mental well-being. Take time for activities that relax and rejuvenate you, such as taking baths, practicing mindfulness, spending time with loved ones, or engaging in hobbies. By prioritizing self-care, you enhance your overall resilience and self-control.

Boosting self-control is a key component of overcoming sugar addiction. By setting clear goals, developing awareness and mindfulness, practicing delayed gratification, building a supportive environment, utilizing cognitive restructuring, implementing stress management techniques, developing healthy coping mechanisms, practicing self-reflection, prioritizing sleep, and engaging in self-care, you can empower yourself to break free from the cycle of sugar addiction.

Remember that self-control is a skill that can be strengthened with practice and consistency. Stay committed to your goals, be patient with yourself, and celebrate every small victory along the way.

With a renewed sense of self-control, you can make empowered choices, nurture your well-being, and build a healthier and more balanced relationship with food. Embrace the journey and step into a life of greater freedom and well-being, free from the grip of sugar addiction.

Chapter Four
Long-Term Solutions

Breaking free from sugar addiction requires long-term solutions that go beyond temporary fixes. By implementing sustainable strategies and making lasting changes to your lifestyle, you can establish a healthier and more balanced relationship with food. In this section, we explore key long-term solutions that can support you on your journey to overcoming sugar addiction.

1. Embrace a Whole-Food, Nutrient-Dense Diet: Shift your focus towards a whole-food, nutrient-dense diet that prioritizes fresh fruits and vegetables, lean proteins, whole grains, and healthy fats. These foods provide essential nutrients, fiber, and satiety, reducing the need for sugary treats. Aim for a well-rounded and varied diet that nourishes your body and supports your overall health.

2. Practice Moderation: Rather than adopting a restrictive mindset, practice moderation and balance in your approach to food. Allow yourself to enjoy occasional treats in controlled portions, without feeling guilty. By practicing moderation, you avoid feelings of deprivation and reduce the likelihood of binge-eating or falling back into old habits.

3. Develop Healthy Habits: Focus on developing healthy habits that promote a sustainable lifestyle. This includes regular meal planning, mindful eating, cooking at home, and practicing portion control. Establishing these habits creates a solid foundation for making healthier food choices and reduces the reliance on sugary foods as a source of comfort or reward.

4. Enhance Food Awareness: Cultivate a deeper awareness of the nutritional content and ingredients in the foods you consume. Read labels, educate yourself about hidden sugars, and make informed choices based on the nutritional value of the foods you consume. This awareness empowers you to make conscious decisions and reduces the consumption of hidden sugars.

5. Foster a Supportive Social Circle: Surround yourself with a supportive social circle that encourages and reinforces your healthier choices. Engage in activities and spend time with friends and family members who share similar health goals. Supportive relationships provide accountability, motivation, and a sense of belonging, making it easier to sustain long-term changes.

6. Continuous Learning and Growth: Stay curious and committed to continuous learning about nutrition, wellness, and the effects of sugar on the body. Attend workshops, read books, listen to podcasts, or consult with professionals to deepen your knowledge and stay motivated on your journey. The more you understand about sugar addiction and its impact, the better equipped you are to make informed choices.

7. Regular Physical Activity: Incorporate regular physical activity into your routine. Exercise not only supports physical health but also contributes to mental well-being and stress reduction. Engaging in activities you enjoy, such as walking, dancing, or practicing yoga, helps to distract from cravings, boost mood, and increase overall self-discipline.

8. Seek Professional Support: If you find it challenging to overcome sugar addiction on your own, consider seeking professional support. Nutritionists, therapists, or support groups specialized in addiction can provide guidance, strategies, and accountability to help you navigate the challenges and sustain long-term changes.

9. Practice Self-Compassion: Be kind and compassionate towards yourself throughout the process. Understand that breaking free from sugar addiction is a journey that may have ups and downs. Embrace setbacks as learning opportunities and practice self-forgiveness. Cultivating self-compassion allows you to maintain a positive mindset and stay motivated on your path to long-term success.

Long-term solutions are crucial for overcoming sugar addiction and maintaining a healthier lifestyle. By embracing a whole-food diet, practicing moderation, developing healthy habits, enhancing food awareness, fostering a supportive social circle, engaging in continuous learning, prioritizing physical activity, seeking professional support when needed, and practicing self-compassion, you can create a sustainable relationship with food.

Remember that the journey is unique to you and requires patience, commitment, and resilience. Embrace the process and celebrate each step forward, no matter how small. With these long-term solutions, you can break free from the grip of sugar addiction, nurture your body and mind, and enjoy a life filled with balanced, nourishing choices.

Empower yourself to live a healthier and more vibrant life, free from the detrimental effects of sugar addiction. You have the power to make lasting changes and create a future filled with well-being and vitality.

Lifestyle Changes

Overcoming sugar addiction requires more than just short-term solutions. It calls for lifestyle changes that support your physical, mental, and emotional well-being. By making intentional shifts in various aspects of your life, you can create a solid foundation for long-term recovery and a healthier relationship with sugar. In this section, we explore key lifestyle changes that can contribute to your journey of breaking free from sugar addiction.

1. Prioritize Nutrient-Dense Foods: Turn your attention to a diet rich in nutrients that will fuel your body. Include a lot of fresh produce in your meals, along with whole grains, lean proteins, and healthy fats. While decreasing the urge for sugary indulgences, these meals offer important vitamins, minerals, and fiber.

2. Meal Planning and Preparation: Make meal planning and preparation a regular part of your routine. Set aside time each week to plan nutritious meals and snacks, and batch cook whenever possible. Having healthy options readily available reduces the likelihood of turning to sugary foods out of convenience.

3. Mindful Eating: Practice mindful eating by paying attention to your food choices, eating slowly, and savoring each bite. Engage your senses and be present during meals, allowing yourself to fully enjoy the flavors and textures of nourishing foods. Mindful eating helps you cultivate a healthier relationship with food and better recognize your body's hunger and fullness cues.

4. Regular Physical Activity: Incorporate regular physical activity into your daily routine. Find activities you like to do, such as yoga, dancing, jogging, or walking. Regular exercise not only benefits your overall health but also lowers stress and improves mood, which lowers the likelihood that you'll turn to sweet foods for comfort.

5. Manage Stress Effectively: Identify and implement stress management techniques that work for you. This may include practicing mindfulness, deep breathing exercises, meditation, engaging in hobbies, or seeking support from a therapist or counselor. Managing stress effectively reduces the reliance on sugar as a coping mechanism and promotes overall well-being.

6. Get Quality Sleep: Prioritize quality sleep as part of your lifestyle changes. Each night, try to get seven to eight hours of unbroken sleep. A good night's sleep elevates your mood, sharpens your memory, balances your hormones, and lessens your need for sweets.

7. Hydration: Make sure you're well hydrated by consuming enough water throughout the day. Staying hydrated promotes overall health and might assist in reducing unwanted eating and desires that might be interpreted as hunger.

8. Cultivate Healthy Coping Mechanisms: Develop alternative, healthy coping mechanisms to deal with emotions and stress. Engage in activities such as journaling, practicing gratitude, spending time in nature, or pursuing hobbies that bring you joy and fulfillment. Finding healthy outlets for stress and emotions reduces the reliance on sugar for comfort or distraction.

9. Create a Supportive Environment: Surround yourself with a supportive environment that aligns with your goals. Communicate your intentions to friends, family, and coworkers, and ask for their support. Remove or minimize the presence of sugary snacks in your surroundings and replace them with healthier options.

10. Practice Self-Care: Prioritize self-care as an essential part of your lifestyle changes. Engage in activities that nourish your mind, body, and soul, such as taking relaxing baths, practicing self-reflection, engaging in creative pursuits, or enjoying hobbies that bring you joy. Taking care of yourself holistically supports your overall well-being and reduces the desire for sugar as a form of self-soothing.

Lifestyle changes are integral to overcoming sugar addiction and maintaining long-term success. By prioritizing nutrient-dense foods, practicing mindful eating, engaging in regular physical activity, managing stress effectively, getting quality sleep, staying hydrated, cultivating healthy coping mechanisms, creating a supportive environment, and practicing self-care, you can build a foundation for lasting recovery. These lifestyle changes not only support your journey to overcome sugar addiction but also promote overall health and well-being.

Remember, implementing lifestyle changes takes time and patience. Be gentle with yourself and embrace progress over perfection. Each small step you take towards a healthier lifestyle contributes to your long-term success in breaking free from sugar addiction.

By making conscious choices, nurturing your body and mind, and fostering a positive and supportive environment, you can create a sustainable and fulfilling life free from the grips of sugar addiction. Empower yourself to make lasting changes and enjoy the benefits of a healthier and more balanced way of living. You have the strength and determination to embrace a new chapter of well-being and vitality.

Nutrition and Exercise

Nutrition and exercise are two vital pillars that play a significant role in overcoming sugar addiction and establishing a healthier lifestyle. By adopting a nutritious diet and incorporating regular physical activity, you can support your body's overall well-being, reduce cravings, and break free from the cycle of sugar addiction. In this section, we explore the importance of nutrition and exercise in your journey towards overcoming sugar addiction.

1. Nourishing Nutrition

Adopting a nourishing diet is crucial in overcoming sugar addiction. Focus on the following key principles:

a. Whole Foods: Embrace whole, unprocessed foods such as fruits, vegetables, whole grains, lean proteins, and healthy fats. These nutrient-dense foods provide essential vitamins, minerals, and fiber while reducing the need for sugary treats.

b. Balanced Meals: Strive for balanced meals that include a combination of carbohydrates, proteins, and fats. This balance helps stabilize blood sugar levels and prevents sharp spikes and crashes that can lead to cravings.

c. Mindful Eating: Practice mindful eating by paying attention to your hunger and fullness cues, savoring each bite, and enjoying your meals without distractions. This helps you develop a healthier relationship with food and reduces mindless snacking.

d. Sugar Awareness: Be mindful of hidden sugars in processed foods and beverages. Read labels, educate yourself about different types of sugar, and make informed choices to minimize your sugar intake.

2. Regular Physical Activity:

Regular exercise is a powerful tool in overcoming sugar addiction. Here's how it can help:

a. Stress Reduction: Exercise helps reduce stress levels, which is often a trigger for sugar cravings. Engaging in physical activity releases endorphins, improves mood, and promotes a sense of well-being, reducing the need for emotional eating.

b. Blood Sugar Regulation: Physical activity helps regulate blood sugar levels by increasing insulin sensitivity and improving glucose metabolism. This reduces the risk of blood sugar fluctuations and subsequent sugar cravings.

c. Distraction and Focus: Engaging in exercise provides a healthy distraction from cravings and redirects your focus towards positive activities. Whether it's a brisk walk, a workout session, or a sport you enjoy, exercise can help break the cycle of turning to sugar for comfort or reward.

d. Body Composition and Energy: Regular exercise contributes to improved body composition, increased muscle mass, and enhanced energy levels. Feeling stronger and more energized can motivate you to make healthier food choices and reduce reliance on sugary foods for energy boosts.

3. Synergy between Nutrition and Exercise
Recognize the synergistic relationship between nutrition and exercise:

a. Pre-Workout Nutrition: Fuel your body with a balanced meal or snack before exercising to optimize energy levels and performance. Incorporate a combination of carbohydrates for energy, proteins for muscle repair, and healthy fats for sustained energy release.

b. Post-Workout Nutrition: After exercising, replenish your body with a nutritious post-workout meal or snack. Focus on quality protein to aid in muscle recovery and repair, along with carbohydrates to replenish glycogen stores.

c. Hydration: Proper hydration is crucial for both nutrition and exercise. Drink water before, during, and after workouts to maintain optimal hydration levels and support overall well-being.

Nutrition and exercise are integral components of overcoming sugar addiction and maintaining a healthy lifestyle. By prioritizing nourishing foods, practicing mindful eating, engaging in regular physical activity, and recognizing the synergistic relationship between nutrition and exercise, you can create a strong foundation for long-term success.

Embrace the power of nutrition and exercise in supporting your journey towards overcoming sugar addiction, improving your overall health, and achieving a balanced and fulfilling life.

Managing Stress

Stress can often be a significant trigger for turning to sugary foods for comfort or emotional relief. Effectively managing stress is essential in overcoming sugar addiction and creating a healthier lifestyle. By implementing effective stress management strategies, you can reduce the reliance on sugar as a coping mechanism and develop healthier ways to navigate challenging situations. In this section, we explore key strategies for managing stress and breaking free from the cycle of sugar addiction.

1. Identify Stress Triggers: Determine the stressors in your life to start. Consider the circumstances, occurrences, or individuals who frequently add to your stress levels. Knowing your stress triggers helps you create specialized techniques to control and lessen their effects.

2. Practice Mindfulness and Relaxation Techniques: Engage in mindfulness and relaxation techniques to calm the mind and reduce stress. Techniques such as deep breathing exercises, meditation, progressive muscle relaxation, or yoga can help restore a sense of calm and balance in your daily life. Regular practice trains your mind to respond to stress in a more composed and centered manner.

3. Prioritize Self-Care: Self-care is crucial for managing stress and reducing the likelihood of turning to sugar for comfort. Dedicate time to activities that bring you joy and relaxation, such as taking a bath, reading a book, listening to music, practicing a hobby, or spending time in nature. Prioritizing self-care nourishes your mind, body, and soul, providing a healthy outlet for stress.

4. Establish Healthy Boundaries: Learn to set and maintain healthy boundaries to protect your mental and emotional well-being. Clearly communicate your needs and limits to others, and be assertive in protecting your time and energy. Setting boundaries helps prevent overwhelm and reduces stress levels.

5. Develop Healthy Coping Mechanisms: Explore and cultivate alternative, healthy coping mechanisms for managing stress. Engage in activities such as journaling, practicing gratitude, engaging in creative pursuits, or seeking support from friends or professionals. Healthy coping mechanisms provide outlets for stress and prevent the reliance on sugar as a quick fix.

6. Regular Exercise: Regular physical activity is not only beneficial for physical health but also an effective stress management tool. Engaging in exercise releases endorphins, which are natural mood boosters, and reduces stress hormones in the body. Find activities you enjoy and incorporate them into your routine to help alleviate stress and reduce cravings.

7. Practice Time Management: By fostering a sense of control and success, efficient time management lowers stress. Set realistic goals, prioritize chores, and divide bigger tasks into smaller, more manageable steps. By successfully organizing your time, you may reduce stress and avoid feeling overwhelmed, which frequently prompts people to turn to sugar for comfort.

8. Seek Support: Don't be reluctant to ask for assistance when you need it. Reaching out to others can offer helpful insight, perspective, and emotional support in managing stress, whether it's by talking to a trusted friend or family member, getting advice from a therapist or counselor, or joining a support group.

9. Get Sufficient Sleep: Put getting good sleep first in your stress-reduction plan. Each night, try to get seven to eight hours of unbroken sleep. Your body and mind are renewed by getting enough sleep, which also strengthens your ability to cope with stress and lowers your propensity to turn to sugary foods for comfort and vitality.

Effectively managing stress is essential in overcoming sugar addiction and maintaining a healthier lifestyle. By identifying stress triggers, practicing mindfulness and relaxation techniques, prioritizing self-care, establishing healthy boundaries, developing healthy coping mechanisms, engaging in regular exercise, practicing time management, seeking support, and getting sufficient sleep, you can navigate stress more effectively and reduce the reliance on sugar as a coping mechanism.

Empower yourself with these strategies, and remember that managing stress is an ongoing process that requires consistent effort and self-awareness. As you implement these stress management strategies, you will gradually develop healthier responses to stress and reduce the need for sugary foods as a temporary escape.

On this path, keep in mind to be kind and patient with yourself. By prioritizing your well-being and using these tactics, you may create a balanced and satisfying life free from the shackles of sugar addiction. Overcoming sugar addiction and controlling stress go hand in hand. Control your stress, look after yourself, and commit to a better, healthier future.

Seeking Professional Help

Seeking professional help is a valuable and important step in overcoming sugar addiction. While self-help strategies and lifestyle changes are beneficial, the guidance and support of trained professionals can provide additional tools, insights, and accountability to aid in your recovery journey. In this section, we explore the benefits of seeking professional help and how it can enhance your efforts to overcome sugar addiction.

1. Expert Guidance and Knowledge: Healthcare professionals, such as doctors, nutritionists, dietitians, and therapists, possess specialized knowledge and expertise in the field of addiction and behavior change. They can offer a deeper understanding of the underlying causes of sugar addiction, provide personalized recommendations, and help tailor an effective treatment plan to address your specific needs and challenges.

2. Individualized Assessment: Seeking professional help allows for a comprehensive assessment of your physical and mental health, as well as an evaluation of your specific addiction patterns and triggers. Professionals can identify any underlying medical conditions or psychological factors that may contribute to your addiction. This personalized assessment forms the basis for developing a targeted treatment approach.

3. Customized Treatment Plans: Professionals can design personalized treatment plans based on your unique circumstances, goals, and challenges. These plans may include a combination of nutritional counseling, behavioral therapy, cognitive restructuring, support groups, and other evidence-based interventions. A customized approach increases the effectiveness of your treatment and maximizes your chances of long-term success.

4. Accountability and Support: Working with professionals provides a valuable source of accountability and support throughout your recovery journey. They can help you stay motivated, track your progress, and provide guidance during challenging times. Regular check-ins and sessions with professionals create a structured framework that reinforces your commitment to overcoming sugar addiction.

5. Addressing Underlying Issues: The basic causes of sugar addiction are frequently emotional, psychological, or physiological. You can investigate and resolve these underlying problems, such as stress, trauma, emotional eating behaviors, or hormone imbalances, with the aid of professionals. You can address the underlying causes of your addiction and create better coping mechanisms by focusing on and resolving these difficulties.

6. Coping Strategies and Relapse Prevention: Professionals equip you with a toolbox of coping strategies to manage cravings, navigate triggers, and prevent relapse. They teach you practical techniques and skills to deal with stress, emotional eating, and other challenges that may arise along your recovery journey. These strategies empower you to overcome obstacles and maintain long-term success.

7. Supportive Environment: Professional help often comes in the form of group therapy or support groups where you can connect with others facing similar challenges. Being part of a supportive community fosters a sense of belonging, reduces feelings of isolation, and provides encouragement, understanding, and insights from peers who can relate to your experiences.

Seeking professional help is a powerful resource in overcoming sugar addiction. The expertise, guidance, personalized assessment, customized treatment plans, accountability, support, addressing underlying issues, coping strategies, and the supportive environment that professionals provide all contribute to a comprehensive and effective recovery journey.

Embrace the opportunity to work with trained professionals who can offer insights and tools to empower you in your quest to overcome sugar addiction. Remember, seeking help is a sign of strength, and it is an investment in your long-term health, well-being, and happiness.

Conclusion

Overcoming sugar addiction is a journey that requires dedication, commitment, and support. Seeking professional help is a valuable resource that can significantly enhance your efforts to break free from the grip of sugar addiction. The expertise, guidance, personalized assessment, customized treatment plans, accountability, support, addressing underlying issues, coping strategies, and the supportive environment provided by professionals can empower you in your recovery journey.

By collaborating with healthcare professionals, such as doctors, nutritionists, dietitians, therapists, or support groups, you gain access to a wealth of knowledge, tailored treatment approaches, and a supportive network. These professionals offer individualized guidance, help you address underlying factors contributing to your addiction, and equip you with practical tools and coping mechanisms to navigate challenges and prevent relapse.

Remember, seeking professional help is not a sign of weakness but rather a courageous step towards a healthier, more fulfilling life. It shows your commitment to taking control of your well-being and seeking the support you need. Embrace the opportunity to work with professionals, leverage their expertise, and benefit from their guidance and support.

As you embark on your journey towards overcoming sugar addiction, remember to be patient and compassionate with yourself. Change takes time, and setbacks may occur. But with the help of professionals, you can build a solid foundation for long-term success and create a life free from the hold of sugar addiction.

Keep in mind that seeking professional help is just one piece of the puzzle. It is important to combine it with other strategies, such as lifestyle changes, stress management techniques, and healthy coping mechanisms. By taking a holistic approach and utilizing all available resources, you increase your chances of achieving lasting recovery and enjoying a healthier, more balanced life.

You deserve to live a life filled with vitality, well-being, and freedom from sugar addiction. Embrace the support of professionals, harness their expertise, and trust in your own strength and determination to overcome the challenges along the way. With professional help and your unwavering commitment, you can break free from sugar addiction and embrace a brighter, healthier future.